WHAT IS

BRONCHITIS

What Is Bronchitis

Understanding The Bronchitis Symptoms And Curing It

Dr. Linda Levinstin

Contents

What Is Bronchitis

Bronchitis is a very common disease in many parts of the world. Most people would have bronchitis at least once in their entire lifetime. It is an illness which develops after you have a cold or other breathing condition. Throughout your lifetime, you would most probably have it, although you may not be sure what it is called.

Among the symptoms is that your chest would throb in pain. You would cough and it hurts. This is the first symptoms when someone has bronchitis. It may be a common condition, but for some people, it may be even worse. For certain people, bronchitis make them unable to do many things and become a very frequent pain. If you are someone who falls into this category, I'm sure you would want to cure yourself and get your life back. You need to gain the strength in order to completely cure from this illness.

With the right knowledge, you could easily do it. Most bronchitis isn't a hard condition to cure. What you need is just time to enable you to push yourself towards improving yourself and strengthen your body.

This book does exactly that. I would discuss the basic understanding of bronchitis, how it affects your health and ensures that it doesn't affect your life. Learning this will enable you to protect yourself for the long term.

Chapter One: The Reality Of Bronchitis

Before you want to cure yourself of any illness, the most important thing is to first know what it is. You need to understand how this illness grows in your body and what it does to your body over the long term. When you have a better understanding of an illness, it would put you in a better position for spotting the symptoms that you would have and taking the right action before you become sicker.

As the effect of bronchitis is something drastic, you would need to read all that you know before you can cure yourself of it. This book would give you a simplified understanding of the illness to enable a cure easily.

Bronchitis is an illness which happens in your lungs. As a matter of fact, it is a condition which affects the inner walls of your air passage ways to your lungs. Bronchitis has the effect of lining up to become infected and inflamed. This causes various symptoms such as fevers, cough, chills and pains in your chest.

These are the common symptoms of bronchitis which is acute. When you have a respiratory infection, it is very common to have this. When you have this, you may have symptoms which last a few days or even weeks. However, most bronchitis isn't something for long.

If, however, you have bronchitis which relapses over and over again, you should be very concerned about it. It could lead to other serious conditions that would deeply affect your life. Seeks medical attention as soon as you can.

There is a high probability that a smoker would develop chronic bronchitis that those who are likely to get acute bronchitis. You would find later in this book more about chronic bronchitis and what you have to worry about. Nevertheless, you should be aware of the difference between acute and chronic bronchitis.

What Should You Look Out For?

When you have bronchitis symptoms, it is a clear indication that you have bronchitis. It is as simple as that. The moment you have any of these symptoms, it is recommended that you seek a doctor straight away.

The top sign that you have this condition is when you have yellow/gray mucus that comes up when you cough. At times, there would even be green colored mucus. Such mucus is called as sputum. When you have such color mucus, it shows that something is wrong with you. Mucus is something that your body produces because it assists the hydration of the body.

When you cough out mucus, it is because you have built up an infection. Mucus normally just slide down your throat when you swallow your saliva. However, when you have too much mucus, your body needs to remove it. Therefore, it coughs it out.

When a person has bronchitis, the airways become inflamed. This is because they produce a large amount of discolored mucus. The color of the mucus is a good sign that you have an infection. However, many people tend to not realize that they have an infection because we normally swallow the mucus.

Most commonly, people don't have too much mucus in their throats for them to cough it out. This is why you need to realize that you have the possibility of having bronchitis although you don't have much mucus.

Having mucus being coughed out isn't the only sign to look out for. Other additional signs have to be on the lookout. These symptoms include:

- Having constant fever

- Feeling chilly
- A sore throat
- Feeling congested
- Burning sensation on your chest
- A pain in your chest that makes you constricted
- Wheezing or coughing.

The moment you experience any of these, together with the mucus symptom, it is a high possibility that you suffer from bronchitis.

Having Chronic Sinusitis

Many times, people make the mistake of thinking that suffers from bronchitis. When checked by the doctor, they are being diagnosed as having chronic sinusitis instead.

Chronic sinusitis is a condition where the cavities linings, which are the bones around your nose, are infected. It is very easy to confuse this condition with bronchitis because mucus discharge is often common with chronic sinusitis.

Additionally, you would have cough that happens when you try to drain mucus from your throat. This mucus comes from your sinuses which drains your throat.

It may seem that these two conditions come from the same symptoms; you need to notice where the mucus come from as well as the secondary symptoms of it. For a better diagnosis, always seek advice from your doctor.

Having Chronic Bronchitis

Earlier, I have clearly mentioned the difference between acute and chronic bronchitis. This book will show you the differences between each. The symptoms between both are different.

Common symptoms of chronic bronchitis include:

- Cough that sticks with you during the winter months but goes away during the summer
- Cough that sticks with you that comes with sputum
- Feeling breathless although you don't exert yourself
- Mild chest pain
- Clubbed fingers

When you work with your doctor and be honest with him/her, you can better determine if you really have chronic bronchitis. If you are really diagnosed with chronic bronchitis, it is pretty common for you to have this condition over and over again. Therefore, you would need to find assistance so that you get the necessary relief.

If you don't get the right help for your condition, you will face other symptoms that would worsen your condition. Therefore, always look for the assistance of a professional because they would know where you are and how to help you over the long term.

Chapter Two: What Causes Bronchitis

Bronchitis is a very special condition. It is a disease which could be both infectious or not. While most cases of bronchitis happen because of a virus, it is generally the very same type which causes a common cold to happen to most sufferers. There are other causes of bronchitis too.

Another common cause of bronchitis is the pollutants in the air that you are breathing. This may include cigarette smoke, smog and chemicals.

Another factor of why bronchitis happens is because of a disease called GERD or gastro-esophageal reflux disease. This condition happens because the acid that is found in your stomach backs up to your gastro esophageal track.

Occupational bronchitis is a condition when those people work in conditions that are unfavorable for good and clean breathing. The pollutants like dusts or fumes go into the breathing airways and thus cause this illness. It is common that some people's condition cure instantly the moment they stop working in such conditions. Therefore, if you are someone with such condition, you need to change your working condition.

What Causes Chronic Bronchitis

Unlike common bronchitis, the causes of chronic bronchitis are a bit more drastic. When you have this condition, your bronchial tubes walls become thickened to a point that it is considered permanent.

Anyone with this condition would cough every day in order to clear his or her throat. This is especially for chain smokers. Therefore, it is highly recommended for you to stop smoking the moment you realize you have this condition. I know that stopping the smoking habit may be more difficult than it sounds, but it is something that you must do in order to heal from your bronchitis over the long term.

Another common way to gauge that you have chronic bronchitis is such: if you have to cough once every day for a minimum of three months, it is more likely that you have chronic bronchitis.

Smoking is generally known as the major reason of chronic bronchitis, but it's not the only reason. You could also find yourself have chronic bronchitis if you like in an areas which has air pollution which is severe or from other toxic gasses.

The sufferers of chronic bronchitis often develop asthma over the long term as well because of this condition. Because of the inflammation over the long term, it blocks the passageways. You would need to talk deeper to your doctor about it.

At Risk Of Acute Bronchitis?

Anyone could possibly get acute bronchitis when they have a cold. Therefore, it seems rational to believe that everyone could be at risk when it comes to developing this condition. However, there are other reasons why this condition could affect you more than other people.

Those who live in a house where there is a smoker would have an increased chance of developing bronchitis. The children living in such arrangements too are commonly known to be more susceptible to this illness. Those who live in terrible conditions like smoking home would also have an increased chance of developing other respiratory infections, colds, asthma or pneumonia.

Besides, there are other conditions which you could possibly end up with if you suffer from bronchitis. These include:

- **GERD** has been discussed in the beginning chapters and it is another reason you experience bronchitis. Known as Gastro Esophageal Reflux

Disease, you are more at risk of bronchitis when you suffer from this. The backup of acids that is created from this cough is a stimulus towards the bronchitis condition.

- Another major risk comes from a **low resistance level**. A person that has low resistance level due to another medical condition they are facing would find it hard to deal with bronchitis.

- Having chronic bronchitis is also a major concern. People who are **exposed to irritants** while working or doing other things regularly have more possibilities of suffering from bronchitis.

If you find yourself having any of these risk factors, you should look for ways to protect yourself. However, if you are already exposed to it and have developed bronchitis, you need to look for way to cure it.

In many cases, especially those that have to do with occupational bronchitis, simply removing the irritants from your daily life would improve your life's quality already. By putting yourself in a better place, you are able to minimize the impact of your surroundings on your health.

However, in many cases when the damage is already permanent, there are more that you would need to do. The best possible way is to stop the damage done before it gets worst.

Finding A Doctor

Although a doctor may help you with curing your bronchitis, if you are an avid reader and understands your illness well, you may not even need one.

However, the decision as to whether you need a doctor lies in you. Depending on the type and severity of your condition, you have to decide on yourself. Of course, if you find yourself suffering too much, then you would definitely need to find a doctor.

When you have acute bronchitis, it is something that even the doctor wouldn't be able to cure it for you. Acute bronchitis is something that you would need to give it time because after some time, it would go away. Normally this would be from a few days to a week or more.

To ensure a speedier recovery, you should get more rest and drink a lot of water. This is perhaps as simple as it gets. When you fill yourself with water, you minimize the possibilities of other irritants stimulating the bronchitis. Another great way to do this is to keep your home's surrounding air moist.

For some people, they may be in such great discomfort that they can't sleep. If they are in such a position, then it is recommended that they see a doctor. The doctor would be able to prescribe the appropriate medication for you to take to help lessen the pain and improve your overall well-being.

Although with the right measure you could cure bronchitis on your own, you should be on the lookout for fever. Fever is something that you should lookout for, but if your temperature reaches above 101 degrees

Fahrenheit, seeing a doctor is an absolute must.

This is additionally important if you find yourself coughing out mucus or blood. Your condition may have regressed terribly. As your bronchitis situation gets worst, you may find yourself having pneumonia. Pneumonia is a very serious condition that may cause death if not treat rightly.

Another factor that determines if you must see a doctor is if your bronchitis situation is longer than a month. Someone who faces chronic bronchitis could also develop other conditions like asthma when their air passageways become inflamed.

Some people should seek a doctor regardless of where they are. The moment you realize that you have bronchitis, don't look to cure it on your own unless you are really certain about what you are doing. You should also be aware of the difficulties that you need to face if you have other chronic health problems like chronic lung problems, congestive heart failure or even asthma.

Anyone who suffers from such chronic problems would be at an increased risk for other healthy complications if bronchitis is allowed to develop.

If you have been having bronchitis for a long period of time, you should definitely seek a doctor. Many people think they could just cure themselves when the situation is more severe than they thought. If your situation has been too long, it may be a sign that you are developing chronic bronchitis. This is especially so for those people who are working in areas where irritants are a main concern.

For those who have such symptoms, you need to look for a doctor. This book gives you a mere understanding of your situation. Because different situations require different treatment, the advice in this book is a mere generalization. If you want a longer term cure, a doctor would help you better.

Chapter Three: What Can Your Doctor Help You With

If you have decided to seek help from a doctor, there are many things that you need to keep in mind. In the previous chapter, I shared about the different situations you would face when dealing with bronchitis.

The Diagnosis

Your doctor would listen to your chest to determine the possibility of you having bronchitis. When he listens to your chest, he is able to determine what is happening inside. He would know if there is mucus build up.

Additionally, he/she would do a chest x-ray which shows the inflamed and enlarged air passageways that would most probably be the problem.

Some doctors would also use a sample of your mucus to determine the type of bronchitis that you have. This sample will determine the amount of bacteria found in the sputum during your cough. Someone who suffers from chronic bronchitis would also need additional testing for the doctor to better understand the situation you are in. A series of tests would be done and your symptoms would be taken into account.

To perform this, a pulmonary function test (PFT) is done. This test would be a requirement for most bronchitis testing. You would be told to blow into the device (known as a spirometer). This would help determine how much air your lungs have after you take a deep breath and blown it out. It is a very simple test and takes only a couple of minutes to be performed. If you are someone who has had several bouts of bronchitis in the past year, this is a test that you must insist on having. There is a high possibility that you have chronic bronchitis.

From these tests, your doctor would be able to know better if you have bronchitis or not. If you are diagnosed with bronchitis, treatment is an absolute must. The level of severity of your illness together with the likeliness of the treatment of it would be determined by him/her. An honest discussion as to your condition is therefore imperative.

Common Treatment From Your Doctor

The moment you have been diagnosed as having bronchitis, the doctor should start the treatment for you. However, for situations of acute bronchitis, there isn't as many treatment as you wish for. As a matter of fact, treatment may not even be a viable option because it is a virus. You would need to allow your body to fight it naturally. Viruses don't go away with any antibiotics.

The way to treat bronchitis is through time and allowing you to naturally take a rest. As a matter of fact, the cure for bronchitis isn't expensive like other chronic illness. It involves:

- **Drinking A Lot Of Fluid.** When you increase the consumption of fluid, you are able to aid in restoring the liquid that you lose during the excessive mucus discharge.

- **Rest.** This is perhaps the most important. When you have bronchitis, you tend to be very tired because of your lungs have to work harder. Taking a good day sleep and don't do too much strenuous work.

- **Medication.** Certain medications that help you stop the cough helps. You would need to ask your doctor for them and understand why you are taking it. There has been some debate about this throughout the years. Many doctors believe that taking medications to suppress your cough isn't something good for the long term. Cough allows you to remove the mucus from your body. Speak to your doctor about it.

If your doctor insists that you take medication, you should always look to take the right one. You may need to inform your doctor of allergies or sickness that you have on a regular basis so that he/she can decide how you should be taking the medication.

Ensure that you also read the labels well to know the content of your medication. It is also important for you to take the right medication between the night and day time ones. This is because you want to ensure that you get the rest you need. You wouldn't want to be taking the day medicine and keep you awake.

You could also ask your doctor about the possible prescription of antibiotics. If you have a bacterial infection which causes the conditions that you are having, antibiotics play a possible role in helping to control.

Sufferers who have problems with chronic lung disorders normally need such help. Those that live in a home with a smoker would also need antibiotics to assist in reducing the seriousness and possibility of developing an infection.

Should your doctor decide that you have asthma, or that you have a high likelihood of developing asthma, the doctor may decide to give you additional treatment for your condition. If it is so, the doctor would need an inhaler in case of emergency and other asthma medication.

They would help in reducing the inflammation in your air passageways. It would also help open them up to allow better passage to your lungs. These things are very important when you have asthma.

With the tests, your doctor could normally describe the proper treatment for you. However, you still need to update him/her about your condition to ensure that the treatment is appropriate.

In most cases, sufficient rest and plenty of fluid intake would be enough to ensure a speedy recovery. Take it as a sign to take a rest when you are diagnosed with bronchitis. Don't push yourself too much.

Chapter Four: Danger Of Not Getting Treatment

The severity of bronchitis is different for different people. For many people, bronchitis may seem like spending a few days resting and losing a bit of weight, but for others, it could lead to various other complications over a lifetime.

The lesser of the problem, acute bronchitis, wouldn't lead to much complication over the long term. This form of bronchitis follows a cold or respiratory condition. To cure this, you would need some prescription medication or simply a visit to the doctor.

However, for people who are weaker, acute bronchitis can prove to be a larger problem than initially thought. It would lead to complications that may be difficult for you to deal with. For older people who have it, it could even lead to a serious case of pneumonia. This is also a concern for smokers. Smokers not only put their life at risk, but also put the lives of their loved ones at risk too.

Therefore, infants and older people are advised to not be around smokers as it would severely complicate the situation. Anyone who suffers would need immediate medical attention so they could be monitored and treated instantly. In more severe cases, hospitalization may even be required.

Frequent Bronchitis

Bronchitis is something which some people deal on a regular basis. For such individuals, bronchitis may even become a norm in their day to day lives. It doesn't seem to go away but just lessen in its seriousness. This is known as chronic bronchitis. Should this happen to you, you need to be aware of it and seek for professional help to maintain your health over the long term.

You should be aware that chronic bronchitis is no laughing matter. It is an indication that something is terribly wrong with your body and treatment is required. It could indicate that you are suffering from asthma or other lung disorder.

In fact, it has been proven that those who suffer from bronchitis has a higher possibility of suffering from lung cancer over the long term.

Lung cancer is the top killer when you smoke. Besides, you are not only killing yourself but also the people close to you. The people who inhale the smoke become victims of the smoke as well. Being exposed to it over a certain period put the inhaler at risk.

It is without a doubt that chronic bronchitis is a condition that seriously impacts your life. When you realize you have this condition, there are many things that you can't do. You would suffer from breathlessness and it may seem that you cough almost all the time. This would cause you to feel sickly for the better parts of your life.

However, with the proper form of treatment from your doctor, you would be able to side track the complications. If you are one of those people who suffer incessantly from this illness, seeing a doctor is perhaps the most important thing right now. It may not seem like such a big deal to you, or you may even get used to it, but it may affect you in the long term. Trust the doctor to provide you with the right treatment over the long term.

Chapter Five:
Understanding COPD

Chronic bronchitis is a disease which has to do with your lungs. When you have chronic bronchitis, coupled with emphysema, you have what is known as Chronic Obstructive Pulmonary Disease (COPD).

This is an important condition to understand as many people are unaware of such a condition. First of all, you need to understand what emphysema is.

Emphysema is a condition that has to do with the lungs and causes the shortness of breath. Coupled with chronic bronchitis, it would cause tremendous problems to the sufferer. Even death.

You could have both of them at the same time. To understand the severity of this condition, I would share some statistics on this disease.

- 20% of those who get COPD gets it from their work environment.
- Female smokers are at more possibility than men to get COPD.
- Victims of air pollution have a higher chance of getting COPD.
- COPD claims the death of more than 120 thousand deaths every year in the United States.
- Smokers have a 80 to 90 % higher risk than those who don't smoke.

The biggest risk that many people are unaware of is that they are under-diagnosed by it. When a person is under-diagnosed, it becomes very dangerous. According to estimates, more than 10 million people in the United States suffer from either emphysema or chronic bronchitis. Imagine that most of them are under-diagnosed. If they were to be diagnosed for the other condition, it would make their condition critical.

When You Have Chronic Bronchitis

The moment you have chronic bronchitis, it is a tough situation to be in. You would feel an inflammation in your bronchial tubes. Your bronchial tubes are your air passageways. They are important in providing clear air for your entire body.

When you have your first bouts with chronic bronchitis, the symptoms would be similar to those that face acute bronchitis.

There would be a heavy discharge of mucus from your coughs and it is a good sign that you have chronic bronchitis.

Your doctor would determine if there is something wrong that causes your bronchitis. Some of them can be from a previous condition that you have or the occupational hazards in your workplace.

During your bronchitis bout, your bronchial tubes would become inflamed and swollen. When this happens, the tubes lining becomes scarred. At time passes, the heavier irritation becomes more problematic as more mucus would be produced. The tubes lining becomes thickened because of this scarring.

From here, your cough becomes more and more painful. Excessive mucus and scarring would lead to other problems with the air flow.

You wouldn't be able to breathe as easily as you could. From here, the progression would get worse until your lungs become scarred as well.

Subsequently, there would be added bacteria in your lungs and tubes. This would be perfect for the bacteria to breed and eventually cuts off the airflow to your lungs. It would cause death.

This is the reason why many people die each year from chronic bronchitis.

Chronic Bronchitis Takes Time To Develop

One thing you need to understand about chronic bronchitis is the fact that it doesn't happen overnight. It is a condition which happens over time and gets worse as time passes. It is a condition that could be treated and cured, given time.

From this next chapter, you would understand how to prevent and improve the life circumstances that you are in when you have bronchitis. However, the problem is that many patients don't go to doctor until bronchitis reaches a severe state. When this happens, the condition would get worse.

Because of the belief that bronchitis is treated as something not serious, many people mistakenly avoid seeing a doctor. They think that they could just cure it themselves. However, bronchitis has to be treated as something which is dangerous and there is a high possibility that it would be a very life-threatening condition.

Don't wait until your condition is in the advanced stage for you to see a doctor. By then, your lungs would already be scarred and injured. By the time you reach this stage, you may even have to deal with other problems like difficulty in breathing and even heart problems. However, like it is said, many things can be prevented from worsening when you take the advice of the doctor.

About Emphysema

The COPD condition is something which is shared by both chronic bronchitis and emphysema. The patients of COPDD would have one or the other. When diagnosed with such a condition, the problem is because of the alveoli inside the lungs.

The alveoli is a location inside your body which absorbs oxygen from the air you breathe and exchanges it to carbon dioxide inside the blood.

The alveoli has very thin and soft walls. Once these walls are damaged, they can't be fixed and it's hard to replace or reverse the damage done to them. From here, small holes would develop in the tissues, especially at the lower lungs. Your body needs them to provide oxygen to the body and remove carbon dioxide from your blood. Therefore, you need to keep them in good condition. Or not, it would become useless and stop functioning all together.

When they are slowly destroyed in such a manner, your body would less likely get the oxygen you need to get into the bloodstream. You would find it hard to get enough air and it leaves you breathless. This is why you find yourself breathless most of the time. From here, you lose the elasticity in your lungs. Your lungs would lose the ability to stretch and come back into shape.

Should this occurs, the body would struggle to keep your airways open enough for your body to have a healthy amount of air. When this happens, you would have great problems trying to exhale and get the air you need for your body.

From here, you can clearly see how frightening this condition is. When these two conditions are together, it can be a tremendously terminal illness. Similar to chronic bronchitis, emphysema takes time to develop too. It happens very slowly too, giving you the idea that isn't something serious.

It is a double-edged sword. When it takes slow to develop, you would think that it isn't that serious. However, it also means that you are able to take more time to improve your condition.

The major cause of emphysema is through the constant exposure of cigarette smoke. It could take several years to develop this sort of severity and during this period, you would be exposed to smoke as a smoker or even second-hand smoker. The majority of those diagnosed are over 45 years old. More than half of them are males (around 60%).

If you find yourself having emphysema, you would develop the cough and shortness of breath. This means that you would find it difficult to do any exercise whatsoever.

You need to talk with your doctor about your condition, your PFT results and extensive X-Rays to determine your condition about the problem.

Chapter Six: Surviving COPD

The key to surviving both chronic bronchitis and emphysema is to get help as soon as you realize that you have any symptoms. This is an important point that you must always remember.

The moment you realize you have most of the symptoms, you need to seek your doctor's help and get the right tests. Should you experience bronchitis more than twice a year or you're a chain-smoker, this is an absolute must. To treat this condition, you need to take several things into consideration.

- **Using Medications**. To put it into perspective, there is no permanent cure for chronic bronchitis or emphysema. Once your lungs have been damaged, it is almost impossible to reverse the damage that has been done on your lungs and bronchial tubes.

Medications that are used to treat chronic bronchitis are used to slow the deterioration in your lungs. This prevents the disease from progressing as fast as it would without medication. In truth, medications are mainly used to treat the symptoms like the coughs that you have and other complications that you may suffer from.

- **Medicating The Symptoms.** To provide you with relief, the doctor would most probably provide you with bronchodilator type medications. These medications would help you relax your bronchial tubes and allow air passageways to open up. This allows for better air flow through them. Such medications are extremely important to keep you symptom-free or lessen the intensity of the symptoms.

- **Should You Take Antibiotics?** Antibiotics are a form of medication that would help deal with your pain. However, you have to bear in mind that acute bronchitis isn't affected by the use of antibiotics because antibiotics doesn't do much to viruses. You could still use antibiotics if there is a secondary infection or to prevent other symptoms from happening.

- **Quality Of Life Deteriorates**. This is perhaps the largest factor that those who suffer from both the illness. As it moves from being just a mere cough to its advanced stages, it becomes harder to do the things that you love doing. At the beginning, you struggle to catch your breath.

Then, you may even need an oxygen supplement and you would eventually need a mechanical respiratory for your daily activities. Anyone who suffers from this condition would struggle to exert themselves physically. They wouldn't be able to do their daily chores or engage in many social activities.

- **Glucocorticosteriods** is another treatment option for those suffering from such conditions. By taking it systematically, you would be able to control bronchitis over the long term.

However, this treatment is still being experimented but it has shown to provide a certain progress towards helping relief from symptoms and slow the progression of bronchitis. This illness is something used only when a patient reaches the acute case. It should be noted though that these medications shouldn't be used for a long period of time because of the side effect.

- **Vaccines.** If you suffer from chronic bronchitis or emphysema, you would need to take flu and pneumonia once a year as it would help keep the illnesses at bay. It would help reduce the symptoms and conditions that you face.

- **Transplantation** is another option when your lungs are damaged. Over the last few years, lung transplantation has been shown to bring tremendous improvements over the past few years.

Anyone who suffers from bronchitis has some chance of qualifying from such treatment. You should note, however, that it isn't for everyone. People who suffer from problems due to the complications arising from the exchange of gasses in their lungs wouldn't do well with lung transplantation and it isn't a viable option for everyone who suffers.

All these factors play an important role in curing your bronchitis. However, you need to be aware that there are many other choices available to someone who suffers from both the illness.

The great way is to improve your health by improving your lifestyle. If you visit your doctor early enough, you are able to better cure your illness.

Chapter Seven: Pulmonary Rehabilitation

Pulmonary rehabilitation is a form of treatment that exists to deal with chronic bronchitis. It deals with restoring and preventative care for individuals that are suffering. The treatment is designed to be customized to fit every patient's needs and the different situations that they face. There isn't any set treatment process but it is something that allows you to take better care of yourself over time.

When your lungs become less capable of providing oxygen at the right quantity to your body, you would subsequently need increased amount of training in order to handle and improve your ability to manage such a progression. Do note that this progression isn't something that you take lightly. During this rehabilitation, your doctor would need to assess you to determine your needs. By then, you would be working on a well-worked program which provides you with several elements.

From skill training, physical reconditioning to psychological support; you would get all of them in order to cope with your current condition. There would also be goals that are created in order for your doctors to determine what you need to improve over time. These goals work as milestones.

Be sure that you are not alone in this process though. You have your friends and family to provide you with the encouragement you need. They are great pillars should you need someone to lean on.

What Is The Therapy Like

Pulmonary rehabilitation includes such following treatments and tools which help aid you in improving your physical health and general well-being.

- Learn how to keep your energy and not waste it throughout the day.
- Learn about how your biology is and what causes this lung disease. You need to learn about the different stages of the disease as well.
- Learn the right hygiene techniques to assist your bronchial tubes, which help provide the added airflow through the passageways.

- Work with your doctors to understand your medical test. Understand what your treatment would be and what you would need to do next.

- Learn how to assess your condition. Learn to spot when you need to seek medical attention and understand what your daily needs are.

- Follow an exercise regimen and learn other techniques that would help you. This may include the right way to breathe, endurance, flexibility and strength training.

- Understanding your medication. You would learn about how your medication works and what it does. This may include all medications from over-the-counter, herbal remedies. You also learn how those medications would have side effects on your body. When you start to learn how important those medications are to you,

you would be more consistent with your medication intake.

- Environmental control is also important. You need to remove any pollutants from your house that would make your condition worse over time. You will need to understand what stimulates your infection as well.

Additionally, you would learn other tools which help you improve your daily living. Managing sleep disturbances like insomnia and sleep apnea is also important because many of those situations can be incredibly stressful and uncomfortable.

Without a doubt, lung diseases like this create a strain on your sexual intimacy. You need to learn to stop smoking. Improving your nutrition and getting constant exercise is also incredibly important.

Travelling can also be difficult for someone who has this disease. You need to learn how to travel despite the illness and how to improve your daily methods of coping with this illness. You wouldn't want it to impact too much of your daily activities. Learning how to manage stress when it comes is also important.

For most patients it is important to place a priority on learning how to breathe well. Using your oxygen well is important because when you use it well, it aids your body in improving your condition.

Pulmonary Rehabilitation Purpose

Although it may seem like it takes a lot of work to create such an intensive care package, it does make a lot of difference in your life. With pulmonary rehab, you are in the best position to deal with your condition. This also depends a lot on which stage you are in to gain back your quality of life.

It has been shown that pulmonary rehabilitation is beneficial to improve your physical strength and ultimately allows you to perform your daily activities. You would find doing your daily activities much easier than previously.

One of the most crucial things towards improving your quality of life is to have the right education. If you take the time to educate yourself and understand what you need to do, you learn what it takes to improve your condition.

This is what the rehabilitation program focus on: Improving your quality of life. Besides, pulmonary rehabilitation could also help improve survival in patients who have lung disease or chronic bronchitis.

While a complete cure from the condition is unlikely, it would definitely improve your survival hopes and improve your quality of life over time. You would also find improvements such as:

- You can return to work.
- You would feel stronger throughout the day.
- Learn more about the situation you are in.
- You can perform other sporting activities.
- Improve your respiratory symptoms.
- Reduce the dependency you have on medical care.

You need to remind yourself that your condition is unique. You need to deal with it differently as you find fit.

However, you also need to know that pulmonary rehabilitation isn't suitable for certain lung diseases like asthma. Although it may not be beneficial for you, this program would help improve your general health. It may not help you directly, but indirectly.

Speak to your doctor about how to use this program. Find out how it could help you over the long term. As you speak with your doctor about the right assessment for your situation, your will know your condition better. The right medical tests and treatment would be provided for you.

As pulmonary rehabilitation is something that can be tailor-made, most patients would generally benefit from it. If you doctor says it wouldn't help you, have a thorough discussion with your doctor to find out why. You could also get a second opinion from another doctor.

You should always be honest with your doctor. Communicate what you need with your doctor. The doctor would be able to provide you with extensive information about your question. Most importantly, you need to know that you are in control your destiny when it comes to dealing with chronic bronchitis.

Chapter Eight: Making Lifestyle Changes

From my experience, the people that are equipped to deal with chronic bronchitis are those who are willing to make the necessary lifestyle changes. Even small lifestyle changes go a long ways towards improving your chances when dealing with it.

From bad habits such as smoking, eating unhealthy and not exercising, you will need to change them in order to stand a better chance of improving your lifestyle. Of course, you could continue doing what you have done all along. If you want your condition to worsen, keep doing what you have been doing all this while. Perhaps, what you are doing all this while is the thing that has put you in this position in the very first place.

Understand that there is no easy way out from it. It would require some sacrifices if you want to improve your health. You need to make very important but difficult decision. There isn't an easy way around it. Needless to say, giving up some of those things that aren't helping you would only improve your survival changes over the long term.

You may be surprised by the fact that just small changes in your lifestyle would go a long way towards increasing your longevity and gives you the strength to go about your daily activities. Because you have damaged your body to such an extent in the past, to change what you have done isn't easy.

In this chapter, you would learn what lifestyle changes that you need to make. They may be simple but extremely important. It may be difficult but with the right effort and the support from the people around you, you may be able to deal with it.

Quality Of Your Air

The air quality of your work area is perhaps something that would affect heavily the condition of your illness. If your work area has poor quality, you have to look to either change it or stop working there all together. You wouldn't want your chronic bronchitis situation to get worse from it already is.

When the air that you surround yourself with is filled with chemicals or other pollutants, they would irritate your breathing and put you in an extremely bad position.

However, if you find it hard to move from that area, you can look to improve the condition that you are in. Look for the reason for the contaminants that are in the air. Reduction of chemical use would also help reduce pollution.

You could also use air purifying tools to help you. There are plenty of air purifiers in the market to clean the air in your surroundings.

Talk to your manager about your condition. Tell him/her that you need to move to a better condition because the condition would heavily affect you over the long term.

However, if your manager is insistent, the only way is to quit your job. You can't put yourself in such a bad position because it would only bring in more harm over the long term. It will only cost more money over the long term.

Smoking

It is without a doubt that smoking is a major cause of chronic bronchitis. You must definitely stop it regardless of what it takes. I know it is easier said than done, but you need to consider the consequences once you stop doing it. This is perhaps the hardest change you would have to make in improving your general well-being.

Should you continue to smoke, you would add more damage to your lungs and bronchial tubes. Over time, you would worsen your condition and push you father through the stages of chronic bronchitis and shutting off your oxygen supply. This would result in feeling breathlessness even doing light activities.

By stopping your smoking habit, you stop putting unnecessary stress on your lungs. You would slow down the progression of chronic bronchitis and would allow your body to repair the damage that has been done. Remember that although the change can be very difficult, the changes it makes to your overall life can be tremendous.

There has been multiple research that are being done to improve your chances of quitting smoking. There are a lot of help that you can use to stop the habit over the long term.

If you want to stop smoking, you need to understand why you depend on them. Speak to your doctor about your habit. Try to understand why you smoke and why it has become an importance in your daily life. Once your doctor better understand your dependency, he or she would give you the right treatment for stopping the habit.

For those who aren't aware of it, you can get help with your smoking habit by calling any smoking hotlines. The doctor would help by prescribing medication. Another great way is to attend support group meetings.

Besides, you can also take pills or patches that reduce your nicotine dependence. Like when you have your nicotine from a patch, you wouldn't do the harm that you will get from smoking. Therefore, patches would prove to be a safer relief than using cigarettes.

If you are someone who have to deal with secondary smoke, you also need to take into consideration how to change your situation. You may need to move to somewhere healthier or find a way to remove the smoke. You should be aware that secondary smoke is as bad for you as it does to the smoker.

Just stop smoking once and for all. It is perhaps the most important criteria towards a long term cure for your chronic bronchitis. If you continue with this smoking habit, you will only put yourself in more harm over the long term.

Alleviating Your Bronchitis Symptoms

When you suffer from any form of bronchitis, you need to make multiple lifestyle changes. They may seem small, but the long term effects are tremendous. Among them include:

- **Make It A Habit To Ask For Help.** Many people who get bronchitis tend to believe that they can cure it themselves. However, it is simply not so. The moment you realize you are not well, seek the help of a doctor when you find your condition is severe.

- **Use A Humidifier.** A humidifier is great as it put moisture into the air, making the air less humid. When you use it while you sleep, you would reduce your coughing tendencies. You could also take a hot shower as the steam would help your body better adapt.

- **Drink A Lot Of Water.** When you have such respiratory infection such as bronchitis, it is important to drink a lot of water. Water helps your body function better over the long term.

- **Get Plenty Of Rest.** When you feel the symptoms of bronchitis coming, you need to take some time to rest. Stop your activities and just relax. You need extra time to sleep. When you start resting and conserving your energy, you allow your body to better deal with the stress from coughing incessantly.

Oxygen Therapy

Oxygen therapy is something is not well known among many patients of chronic bronchitis. If your doctor feels that you need it, you should definitely consider getting it. Oxygen therapy would help improve your quality of life as it helps give your body an increase amount of oxygen to perform your daily functions well.

If you find yourself having problem breathing, this is a treatment that you must definitely consider. People who don't use this therapy if their doctor feels they need it would feel that their daily activities deeply impacted. When the oxygen levels in your body is too low, you will feel tired very fast. You may even pass out or slip into a coma.

This therapy is done through the use of a nose piece and a tank. Although this therapy is used in more severe situations, it is something very common nowadays among bronchitis sufferers. It gets a great amount of oxygen into your blood quickly, thus improving the quality of your blood circulation.

Summary

In summary, these practices would help improve your health over the long term. If you take the time and effort to implement it, you can be sure that your lifestyle would be changes for the better over the long term. You need to learn to be honest to yourself and how serious are you about curing your bronchitis.

If you are really serious, then you would definitely put in the required effort. Always follow your doctor's orders. Learning all you can about your condition and the illness that you have is very important.

In short, the changes in your life are as follows:

- Quality of your air
- Smoking

- Alleviating Your Bronchitis Symptoms
- Oxygen Therapy

Chapter Nine: Changing What You Eat

You not only need to follow what your doctor recommends when it comes to curing your condition. You may also need to use a number of alternative treatments or medications to improve your medical condition and quality of life.

The thing about alternative medication is that there isn't a particular method of healing your condition. As different people react differently towards the medication that they take, you wouldn't be sure if your body would be healed just by taking a certain alternative medication.

Another thing to always remember is to ensure that the medication that you take does not cause a chemical effect due to the interaction with other medication that is prescribed. You would have to talk to your doctor about this.

Supplements

Most diets don't have enough nutrients to provide the sufficient nutrition. You should definitely look to consume a diet which has all the nutrients you need. However, different people have different additional needs. Supplements are the answer to it.

It is necessary for you to take extra nutrients to give your body the strength it needs to fight your condition. Eating the right supplements would aid your body in being stronger over time.

The most important nutrient is to take a good quality multi-vitamin. Multi-vitamin are a form of supplement which is packed with nutrients that provide additional supplement to your diet. They are not expensive to take, and you could take it once or twice a day.

For someone who suffers from chronic bronchitis, the common supplement which you must take includes:

- **Zinc.** Important supplement for helping you boost your immune system and help keep viruses at bay. Viruses which cause colds and other respiratory infection could be avoided when you are properly nutrition with zinc.

- **N-Acetyl-Cysteine (NAC)** is very effective in dissolving the mucus in your body. Over time, NAC would improve your symptoms and help you feel better.
- **Vitamin C**
- **Bromelain**
- **Quercetin**

All these supplements would help keep your body healthy. Over time, supplements would ensure that infections and illness are kept at bay.

Additionally, it would also include your body with the right fuel to overcome symptoms and improve the quality of the patient's life. However, you need to take into account how the supplements may affect you. Talk to your doctor about it.

Nutrition

Like it or not, your nutrition plays an important role and directly relates to your body's health. Once you improve your diet, you would subsequently improve your body's strength and its ability to manage stress that you are under.

Firstly, your doctor would determine what nutrition you need. From your cholesterol to your body weight, you need to know what nutrients you lack. If the doctor finds that you need certain nutritional benefits, you should find a way to incorporate it into your life. Among the way you could implement it include:

- **Eat More But Smaller Meals.** You need a balanced meal which is filled with fiber-rich food like fruits and vegetables with other smaller portion of protein like meat.

- **Work Out A Meal Plan.** Talk to a professional dietician would encourage a better health and regular well-being. You may even need to lose some weight if the dietician found fit. Ask your doctor to recommend a dietician for you.

- **Drink More Fluids.** When more water is taken in, the extra water would assist the body and cells well-hydrated and reduce the production of mucus.

- **Increase Amount Of Fat.** Fat is something that affects the levels of carbon dioxide production. It will decrease the level of it, thus making it easier for the lungs to pump it out from your body.

- **Increase Vitamins And Minerals Intake.** Like said before, such nutrients assist the body in getting stronger and would help you fight the illness.

- **Stop Consuming Unhealthy Calories**. When you consume unhealthy calories, you gain weight. Over the long run, the weight would make you weaker and less likely to fight the illness.

Without a doubt, you need to improve your general health and well-being to give your body the right and necessary nutrients. If you find it difficult to give up food, start slow. Try to lessen the intake initially and then slowly work your way up towards eliminating them altogether.

The Power Of Herbs

You not only can use diet and supplements to improve the condition of your body, you could also empower your body by taking herbal products. Herbs is something that has been used for a few thousands year to assist in improving a person's well-being.

In this day and time, there is a growing need for herbal solution because of its holistic approach that it would provide your body that conventional medication simply can't. According to market research, more people are beginning to accept that herbs as a great way to improve their well-being. Besides, herbs also have fewer side effects compared to common medications.

Before you start taking any herbal product, you need to talk to your doctor about it. Ask him/her about the possible consequences that would happen when you take herbal products. You need to ensure that it doesn't interact badly with the current medications that you are taking. However, make it a point to not stop your medications without your doctor's approval. These are few herbal products would help you improve your bronchitis symptoms:

- **Eucalyptus** is something that has been known to treat your cough and protect against the production of phlegm. You can get this nutrition from using eucalyptus oil. It would be able to loosen your phlegm over time. You could also get eucalyptus to inhale and provide you with the relief from your common symptoms.

- **Peppermint** is a very good herbal product to treat cough and congestion because it has menthol. It would also assist you in thinning out mucus and relief in phlegm that many patients struggle with.
- **Barberry** is known for its incredible ability to prevent infection. It also has alternative benefits like improving your immune system over time.
- **Slippery Elm** helps you improve if you have sore throat.
- **Stinging Nettle** helps improve a cough as it works as a expectorant which assist in getting phlegm out of your system when coughing.

Although you wouldn't need a prescription to obtain such herbs, you need to be aware of the possible consequences of taking them.

Most of these could be found from your local health food store. You should find for a capable herbologist to decide the right herbal solution for you. They would be able to recommend what it takes to improve your condition and the right amount to take.

Beside herbs, you could also use other form of relief that is beneficial. Many of those reliefs are extremely beneficial, although you wouldn't be able to feel the effects over the short term.

One great method is by using aromatherapy. It is a great way to ensure that you are surrounded by healthy air. You could do it by using a humidifier to release essential oils into the air. This is especially beneficial when you put it at night.

Another method is through the ancient practice of acupuncture. Acupuncture has been known to treat many illnesses. This includes chronic bronchitis. Research has found that acupuncture is a proven method of healing the right nerves over the long term. If you find a skilled acupuncturist, you would be lucky as this is an extremely beneficial treatment.

Although many of these treatments are proven, you have to protect yourself by getting the right knowledge. Talk to your doctor about the possible side effects that would happen on you.

Chapter Ten: Coping With The Psychological Effects Of Bronchitis

From experience, I can definitely say that bronchitis is something which affects you tremendously. This is especially so for those who reach the severe cases of chronic bronchitis.

Their entire lives would be changed because of this illness. I have known a patient who had to quit her job and be completely dependent on her parents for half a year. This is due to the fact that her working environment was very polluted.

She struggled to find for a job and had to move in with her parents while looking for ways to deal with the acuteness of her situation.

Anyone who reaches the chronic stage of bronchitis would pretty much feel down because of the many things that have to stop doing. Even a person's sexual life would be impacted. You would struggle to be as intimate as you once was with your partner. Besides, COPD also often creates sexual problems.

This is especially evident in men. Because their body is weak from the constant coughing, they would struggle with holding on to an erection. Someone who is sexually active all along would struggle to cope with such a change.

You would also need to restrict your mobility because travelling may be something very difficult. If you travel to a place where the air is even slightly polluted, you would struggle to breathe. This is the truth that you have to face once your deal with bronchitis.

That is why it is mentioned multiple times about the important of early detection. Early detection saves you a lot of pain, together with the hassle of stopping your daily activities.

You need to accept the fact that your life isn't what it used to be once you are diagnosed with this disease. Don't be in denial and refuse treatment. You would only put yourself in more harm in the long term.

Chapter Eleven: Bronchitis Can Be Dealt With

Both acute and chronic bronchitis is a very serious condition. It is a condition that would lead to death if not dealt with properly. It would threaten your life. If you don't take the effort to improve your health now, you would have to pay for the consequences in the future. If you do really put in the significant effort, you would be able to make a big change in your life.

In short, acute bronchitis may seem like just a bad cold. However, chronic bronchitis is a severe condition that needs to be differentiated. The only way to ensure that you control the disease is to take action early.

Look to ensure that you catch it early to control its progression. If you do the right thing, you would be able to survive it without any hassle.

If you choose to ignore it, chronic bronchitis can be very fatal. The damage it does to your lungs can't be repaired easily. Even transplantation may not work well for you. That is why you need to take action as soon as your realize you have this condition. Don't let the condition linger.

Don't just read about this condition. Take time to implement the changes needed. Many of them are already mentioned in this book. Speak to your doctor about your condition to work out a plan of treatment for your bronchitis. Also, ensure that you consistently monitor your healthy.

With the right treatment, you would be able to control it and live a healthy life. The power lies in you. If you do, you would live a higher quality life despite suffering from bronchitis.

Resources

Want to cure bronchitis using a method that doesn't depend on prescription antibiotics or costly doctor bills?

Learn how an ex-smoker and chronic sufferer of bronchitis completely eliminated his coughing, phlegm and wheezing using a thousand-year old secret that thousands of bronchitis sufferers have COMPLETELY CURED THEMSELVES FROM... FASTER than they ever imagined.

http://bronchitis.wellbeingvalley.com/

www.ingramcontent.com/pod-product-compliance
Lightning Source LLC
Chambersburg PA
CBHW070544290526
45790CB00002B/589